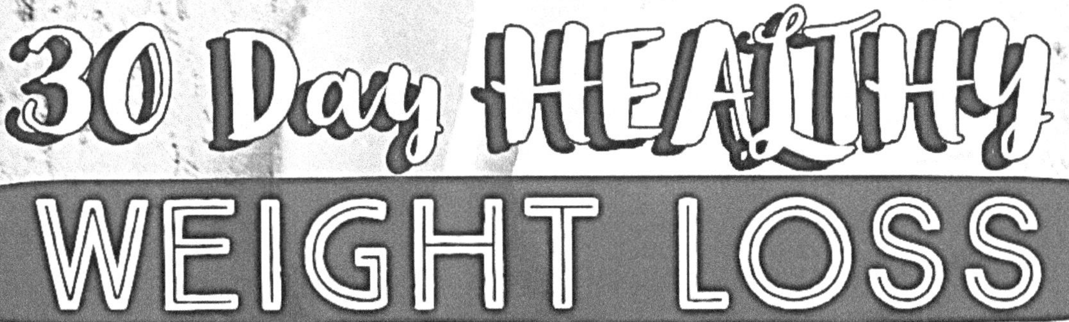

30 Day HEALTHY WEIGHT LOSS Recipes for Seniors

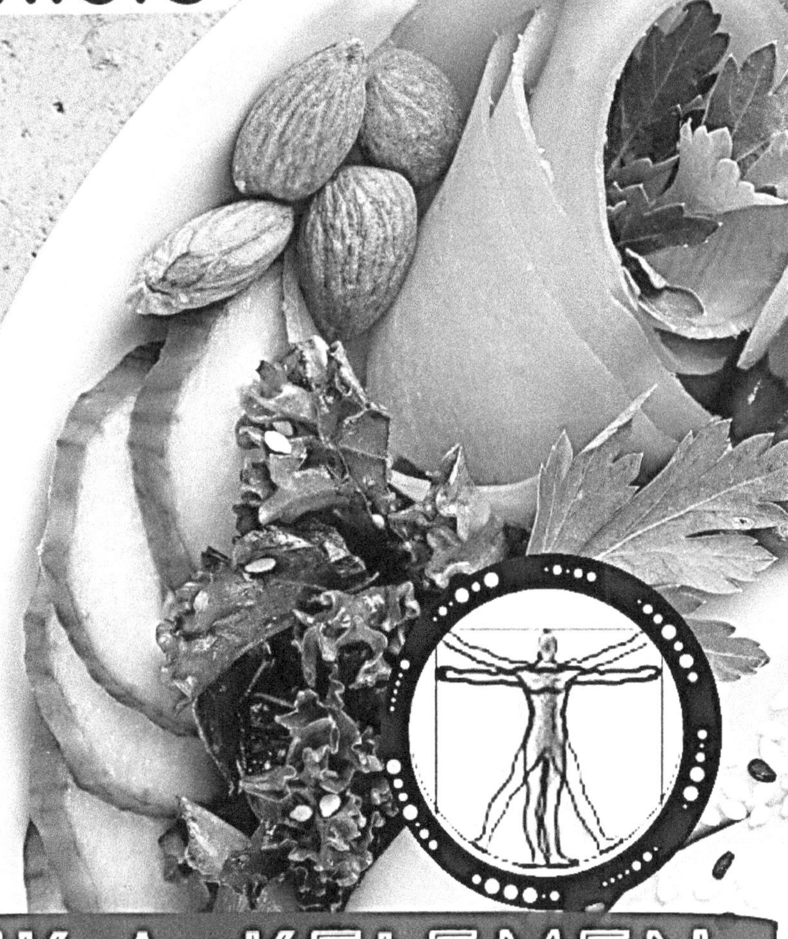

FRANK A. KELEMEN

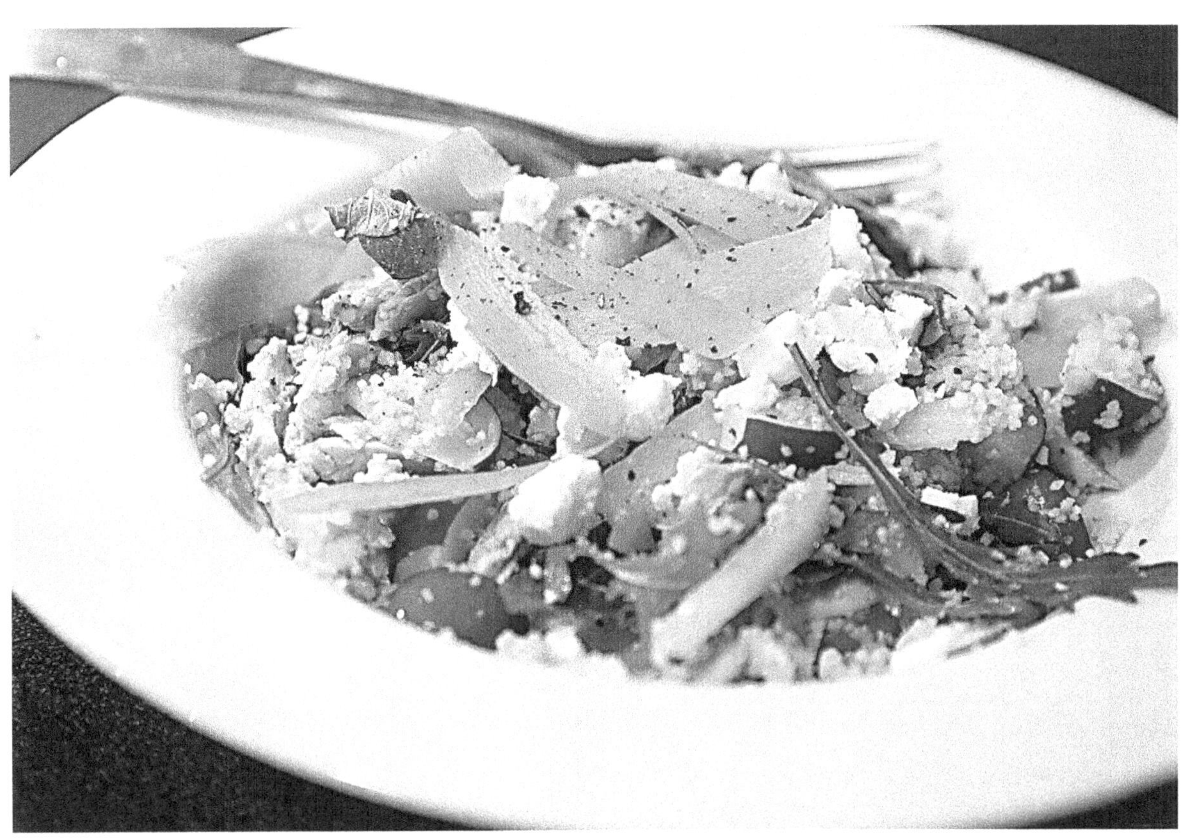

Contents

HEALTHY Weight Loss Recipes

Brain Health Meal Plan for People Over 60

Benefits

1. Cognitive Function Support: The nutrient-rich foods in this plan, particularly those high in omega-3 fatty acids and antioxidants, may help maintain and potentially improve cognitive function, including memory and focus.

2. Reduced Inflammation: The anti-inflammatory properties of foods like fatty fish, leafy greens, and berries may help reduce brain inflammation, which is associated with cognitive decline.

3. Improved Cardiovascular Health: Many of the foods in this plan support heart health, which is closely linked to brain health due to the importance of good circulation for cognitive function.

4. Enhanced Mood: The balanced nutrition provided may help stabilize mood and potentially reduce the risk of depression, which can affect cognitive health in older adults.

5. Better Sleep: Nutrient-dense foods and balanced meals can contribute to improved sleep quality, which is crucial for brain health and memory consolidation.

6. Increased Energy Levels: The steady supply of complex carbohydrates and lean proteins can help maintain consistent energy levels throughout the day.

7. Weight Management: Balanced, portion-controlled meals can assist in maintaining a healthy weight, which is important for overall brain health.

8. Digestive Health: The high fiber content from whole grains, fruits, and vegetables supports digestive health, which is increasingly recognized as important for brain function.

9. Reduced Risk of Chronic Diseases: This nutrient-dense diet may help reduce the risk of chronic diseases like diabetes and hypertension, which can negatively impact brain health.

10. Improved Nutrient Absorption: The variety of foods ensures a wide range of nutrients, and some combinations (like vitamin C with plant-based iron sources) can improve nutrient absorption.

11. Potential Neuroprotective Effects: Antioxidants and certain nutrients in this plan may offer neuroprotective benefits, potentially slowing age-related cognitive decline.

12. Hydration Support: While not explicitly part of the meal plan, the water content in many of the fruits and vegetables supports overall hydration, which is crucial for cognitive function.

13. Sensory Stimulation: The variety of flavors, textures, and aromas in the meals can provide sensory stimulation, which is beneficial for brain health.

14. Social Engagement: Preparing these meals can encourage social interaction if done with family or friends, which is important for cognitive health in older adults.

15. Establishment of Healthy Habits: Following this plan for 30 days can help establish long-term healthy eating habits, providing ongoing benefits for brain health.

Remember, while this meal plan is designed to support brain health, individual results may vary. It's always recommended to consult with a healthcare professional or registered dietitian before making significant changes to one's diet, especially for individuals with existing health conditions.

Rate of Weigh Loss

The rate of weight loss can vary from person to person, but here are typical weight loss data for an average person:

Week 1: 2-4 lbs (0.9-1.8 kg)

Week 2: 1-2 lbs (0.45-0.9 kg)

Week 3: 1-2 lbs (0.45-0.9 kg)

Week 4: 1-2 lbs (0.45-0.9 kg)

Total expected weight loss over 30 days: 5-10 lbs (2.3-4.5 kg).

These numbers are based on general expectations for healthy weight loss. It's important to note that individual results may vary depending on factors such as starting weight, adherence to the diet, exercise intensity, and individual metabolism.

Consistency, patience, and regular monitoring of progress are crucial for sustainable weight loss on the keto diet. It's also essential to consult with a healthcare professional, especially if you have any underlying medical conditions, to ensure the keto diet is appropriate and safe for you.

30 Day HEALTHY Recipes Meal Plan

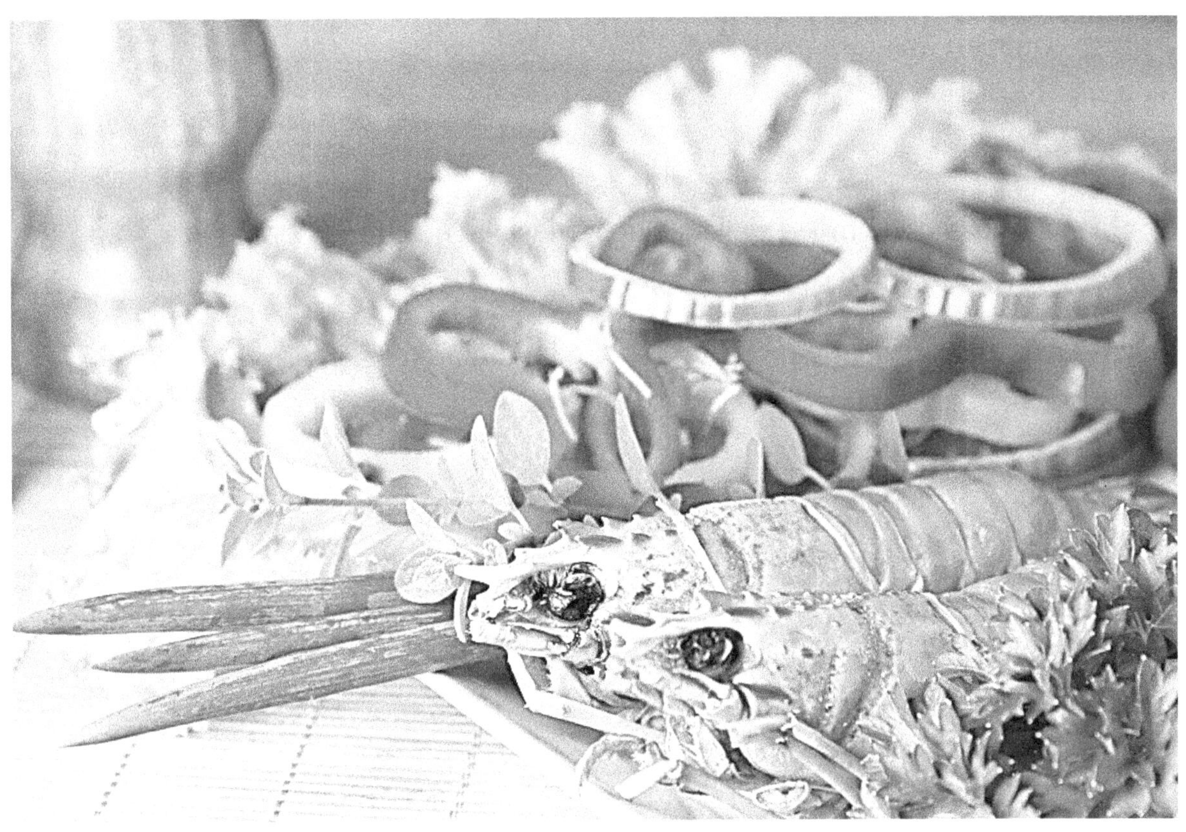

Day 1

Breakfast: Blueberry Walnut Oatmeal

Recipe:

- 1/2 cup rolled oats

- 1 cup unsweetened almond milk

- 1/4 cup fresh blueberries

- 1 tbsp chopped walnuts

- 1 tsp honey

Cook oats with almond milk, top with blueberries, walnuts, and honey.

Macronutrients: 310 calories, 45g carbs, 12g fat, 8g protein

Lunch: Grilled Salmon Salad

Recipe:

- 4 oz grilled salmon

- 2 cups mixed greens

- 1/4 avocado, sliced

- 1/4 cup cherry tomatoes

- 1 tbsp olive oil

- 1 tsp lemon juice

Grill salmon, mix greens with avocado and tomatoes, dress with olive oil and lemon juice.

Macronutrients: 380 calories, 10g carbs, 26g fat, 32g protein

Dinner: Lentil and Vegetable Soup

Recipe:

- 1/2 cup cooked lentils

- 1 cup mixed vegetables (carrots, celery, onions)

- 2 cups low-sodium vegetable broth

- 1 tsp olive oil

- 1 clove garlic, minced

- 1 tsp dried thyme

Sauté vegetables in olive oil, add garlic and thyme. Add lentils and broth, simmer until vegetables are tender.

Macronutrients: 250 calories, 40g carbs, 5g fat, 15g protein

Day 2

Breakfast: Greek Yogurt Parfait

Recipe:

- 1 cup Greek yogurt

- 1/4 cup granola

- 1/2 cup mixed berries

- 1 tbsp chia seeds

Layer yogurt, granola, berries, and chia seeds in a glass.

Macronutrients: 340 calories, 35g carbs, 12g fat, 25g protein

Lunch: Turkey and Avocado Wrap

Recipe:

- 1 whole wheat tortilla

- 3 oz sliced turkey breast

- 1/4 avocado, mashed

- 1 cup spinach leaves

- 1 tbsp hummus

Spread hummus on tortilla, add turkey, avocado, and spinach. Roll and slice.

Macronutrients: 320 calories, 25g carbs, 15g fat, 25g protein

Dinner: Baked Cod with Roasted Vegetables

Recipe:

- 4 oz cod fillet

- 1 cup mixed vegetables (broccoli, cauliflower, bell peppers)

- 1 tbsp olive oil

- 1 tsp lemon juice

- 1 tsp dried dill

Bake cod at 400°F for 15 minutes. Toss vegetables with olive oil and roast for 20 minutes. Season with lemon juice and dill.

Macronutrients: 280 calories, 15g carbs, 12g fat, 30g protein

Day 3

Breakfast: Spinach and Mushroom Omelet

Recipe:

- 2 eggs

- 1/4 cup chopped spinach

- 1/4 cup sliced mushrooms

- 1 oz feta cheese

- 1 tsp olive oil

Sauté mushrooms, add spinach. Beat eggs, pour over vegetables, add feta, and fold.

Macronutrients: 250 calories, 5g carbs, 18g fat, 20g protein

Lunch: Quinoa and Chickpea Salad

Recipe:

- 1/2 cup cooked quinoa

- 1/4 cup chickpeas

- 1 cup mixed greens

- 1/4 cup cucumber, diced

- 1 tbsp olive oil

- 1 tsp lemon juice

Mix all ingredients, dress with olive oil and lemon juice.

Macronutrients: 320 calories, 40g carbs, 15g fat, 12g protein

Dinner: Grilled Chicken with Sweet Potato

Recipe:

- 4 oz grilled chicken breast

- 1 small sweet potato, baked

- 1 cup steamed broccoli

- 1 tsp olive oil

- 1 tsp dried rosemary

Grill chicken, season with rosemary. Serve with baked sweet potato and steamed broccoli drizzled with olive oil.

Macronutrients: 350 calories, 30g carbs, 8g fat, 35g protein

Day 4

Breakfast: Whole Grain Toast with Almond Butter and Banana

Recipe:

- 2 slices whole grain bread

- 2 tbsp almond butter

- 1 small banana, sliced

- 1 tsp chia seeds

Toast bread, spread almond butter, top with banana slices and chia seeds.

Macronutrients: 420 calories, 55g carbs, 20g fat, 15g protein

Lunch: Mediterranean Tuna Salad

Recipe:

- 3 oz canned tuna in water, drained

- 1 cup mixed greens

- 1/4 cup cherry tomatoes, halved

- 1/4 cup cucumber, diced

- 2 tbsp olives, sliced

- 1 tbsp olive oil

- 1 tsp lemon juice

Mix all ingredients, dress with olive oil and lemon juice.

Macronutrients: 300 calories, 10g carbs, 18g fat, 28g protein

Dinner: Stir-Fried Tofu with Brown Rice

Recipe:

- 4 oz firm tofu, cubed

- 1/2 cup cooked brown rice

- 1 cup mixed vegetables (bell peppers, snap peas, carrots)

- 1 tbsp soy sauce (low sodium)

- 1 tsp sesame oil

- 1 clove garlic, minced

- 1 tsp grated ginger

Stir-fry tofu and vegetables with garlic and ginger. Add soy sauce and sesame oil. Serve over brown rice.

Macronutrients: 380 calories, 45g carbs, 15g fat, 20g protein

Day 5

Breakfast: Chia Seed Pudding

Recipe:

- 2 tbsp chia seeds

- 1 cup unsweetened almond milk

- 1/4 cup mixed berries

- 1 tbsp chopped nuts

Mix chia seeds with almond milk, refrigerate overnight. Top with berries and nuts.

Macronutrients: 280 calories, 30g carbs, 18g fat, 10g protein

Lunch: Lentil and Spinach Soup

Recipe:

- 1/2 cup cooked lentils

- 2 cups low-sodium vegetable broth

- 1 cup spinach

- 1/4 cup diced carrots

- 1/4 cup diced onions

- 1 tsp olive oil

- 1 tsp cumin

Sauté vegetables in olive oil, add lentils, broth, and cumin. Simmer, add spinach before serving.

Macronutrients: 250 calories, 40g carbs, 5g fat, 15g protein

Dinner: Baked Salmon with Quinoa and Asparagus

Recipe:

- 4 oz salmon fillet

- 1/2 cup cooked quinoa

- 1 cup asparagus spears

- 1 tbsp olive oil

- 1 tsp lemon juice

- 1 tsp dried dill

Bake salmon at 400°F for 12-15 minutes. Steam asparagus. Serve with quinoa, drizzle with olive oil and lemon juice, sprinkle with dill.

Macronutrients: 420 calories, 30g carbs, 20g fat, 35g protein

Day 6

Breakfast: Vegetable Frittata

Recipe:

- 2 eggs

- 1/4 cup mixed vegetables (spinach, bell peppers, onions)

- 1 oz feta cheese

- 1 tsp olive oil

Sauté vegetables, beat eggs and pour over. Add feta and bake at 350°F for 10-12 minutes.

Macronutrients: 250 calories, 5g carbs, 18g fat, 20g protein

Lunch: Chickpea and Avocado Sandwich

Recipe:

- 2 slices whole grain bread

- 1/4 cup mashed chickpeas

- 1/4 avocado, mashed

- 1 slice tomato

- 1/4 cup sprouts

- 1 tsp mustard

Mash chickpeas with avocado, spread on bread. Add tomato and sprouts.

Macronutrients: 350 calories, 45g carbs, 15g fat, 12g protein

Dinner: Grilled Turkey Breast with Roasted Brussels Sprouts

Recipe:

- 4 oz turkey breast

- 1 cup Brussels sprouts, halved

- 1 tbsp olive oil

- 1 tsp balsamic vinegar

- 1 tsp dried thyme

Grill turkey breast. Toss Brussels sprouts with olive oil, roast at 400°F for 20 minutes. Drizzle with balsamic vinegar and sprinkle with thyme.

Macronutrients: 320 calories, 15g carbs, 12g fat, 40g protein

Day 7

Breakfast: Smoked Salmon on Whole Grain Toast

Recipe:

- 2 slices whole grain bread

- 2 oz smoked salmon

- 1 tbsp cream cheese

- 1/4 avocado, sliced

- 1 tsp capers

Toast bread, spread with cream cheese. Top with smoked salmon, avocado, and capers.

Macronutrients: 350 calories, 30g carbs, 18g fat, 25g protein

Lunch: Spinach and Strawberry Salad

Recipe:

- 2 cups spinach

- 1/2 cup strawberries, sliced

- 1/4 cup walnuts

- 1 oz goat cheese

- 1 tbsp balsamic vinaigrette

Toss all ingredients together, drizzle with vinaigrette.

Macronutrients: 300 calories, 15g carbs, 25g fat, 10g protein

Dinner: Herb-Roasted Chicken with Sweet Potato and Green Beans

Recipe:

- 4 oz chicken breast

- 1 small sweet potato, cubed

- 1 cup green beans

- 1 tbsp olive oil

- 1 tsp dried rosemary

- 1 tsp dried thyme

Rub chicken with herbs, roast at 375°F for 25 minutes. Toss sweet potato and green beans with olive oil, roast for 20 minutes.

Macronutrients: 380 calories, 30g carbs, 12g fat, 35g protein

Day 8

Breakfast: Turmeric Scrambled Eggs with Whole Grain Toast

Recipe:

- 2 eggs

- 1/4 cup spinach, chopped

- 1/4 tsp turmeric

- 1 slice whole grain bread

- 1 tsp olive oil

Whisk eggs with turmeric, scramble with spinach in olive oil. Serve with toast.

Macronutrients: 300 calories, 20g carbs, 18g fat, 20g protein

Lunch: Lentil and Kale Soup

Recipe:

- 1/2 cup cooked lentils

- 1 cup kale, chopped

- 1/4 cup diced carrots

- 1/4 cup diced onions

- 2 cups low-sodium vegetable broth

- 1 tsp olive oil

- 1 clove garlic, minced

Sauté vegetables in olive oil, add lentils, broth, and garlic. Simmer, add kale before serving.

Macronutrients: 280 calories, 45g carbs, 6g fat, 18g protein

Dinner: Baked Trout with Quinoa and Roasted Vegetables

Recipe:

- 4 oz trout fillet

- 1/2 cup cooked quinoa

- 1 cup mixed vegetables (zucchini, bell peppers, onions)

- 1 tbsp olive oil

- 1 tsp lemon juice

- 1 tsp dried oregano

Bake trout at 400°F for 12-15 minutes. Roast vegetables with olive oil. Serve with quinoa, drizzle with lemon juice and sprinkle with oregano.

Macronutrients: 400 calories, 30g carbs, 18g fat, 35g protein

Day 9

Breakfast: Greek Yogurt with Walnuts and Berries

Recipe:

- 1 cup Greek yogurt

- 1/4 cup mixed berries

- 2 tbsp chopped walnuts

- 1 tsp honey

Mix yogurt with berries, top with walnuts and drizzle with honey.

Macronutrients: 320 calories, 25g carbs, 18g fat, 25g protein

Lunch: Spinach and Feta Stuffed Chicken Breast

Recipe:

- 4 oz chicken breast

- 1/4 cup spinach, chopped

- 1 oz feta cheese

- 1 cup mixed salad greens

- 1 tbsp olive oil

- 1 tsp balsamic vinegar

Stuff chicken with spinach and feta, bake at 375°F for 25 minutes. Serve with salad dressed with olive oil and balsamic vinegar.

Macronutrients: 350 calories, 5g carbs, 20g fat, 40g protein

Dinner: Vegetarian Chili with Brown Rice

Recipe:

- 1/2 cup mixed beans (kidney, black beans)

- 1/4 cup diced tomatoes

- 1/4 cup diced bell peppers

- 1/4 cup diced onions

- 1/2 cup cooked brown rice

- 1 tsp olive oil

- 1 tsp chili powder

Sauté vegetables in olive oil, add beans, tomatoes, and chili powder. Simmer for 20 minutes. Serve over brown rice.

Macronutrients: 380 calories, 70g carbs, 6g fat, 18g protein

Day 10

Breakfast: Whole Grain Pancakes with Blueberries

Recipe:

- 1/2 cup whole grain pancake mix

- 1/4 cup blueberries

- 1 egg

- 1/4 cup almond milk

- 1 tsp coconut oil

Mix pancake batter, fold in blueberries. Cook in coconut oil.

Macronutrients: 350 calories, 45g carbs, 15g fat, 12g protein

Lunch: Tuna and White Bean Salad

Recipe:

- 3 oz canned tuna in water, drained

- 1/4 cup white beans

- 1 cup mixed salad greens

- 1/4 cup cherry tomatoes, halved

- 1 tbsp olive oil

- 1 tsp lemon juice

Mix all ingredients, dress with olive oil and lemon juice.

Macronutrients: 320 calories, 20g carbs, 15g fat, 35g protein

Dinner: Grilled Tofu with Stir-Fried Vegetables

Recipe:

- 4 oz firm tofu

- 1 cup mixed vegetables (broccoli, carrots, snap peas)

- 1/2 cup cooked brown rice

- 1 tbsp soy sauce (low sodium)

- 1 tsp sesame oil

- 1 clove garlic, minced

Grill tofu, stir-fry vegetables with garlic. Serve over brown rice, drizzle with soy sauce and sesame oil.

Macronutrients: 380 calories, 45g carbs, 15g fat, 20g protein

Day 11

Breakfast: Avocado Toast with Poached Egg

Recipe:

- 1 slice whole grain bread

- 1/4 avocado, mashed

- 1 poached egg

- 1 tsp olive oil

- Pinch of red pepper flakes

Toast bread, spread with mashed avocado. Top with poached egg, drizzle with olive oil and sprinkle with red pepper flakes.

Macronutrients: 280 calories, 20g carbs, 18g fat, 12g protein

Lunch: Grilled Chicken and Quinoa Bowl

Recipe:

- 4 oz grilled chicken breast

- 1/2 cup cooked quinoa

- 1/2 cup roasted vegetables (zucchini, eggplant)

- 1 tbsp hummus

- 1 tsp olive oil

Grill chicken, serve over quinoa with roasted vegetables. Top with hummus and drizzle with olive oil.

Macronutrients: 400 calories, 30g carbs, 15g fat, 40g protein

Dinner: Baked Salmon with Asparagus and Sweet Potato

Recipe:

- 4 oz salmon fillet

- 1 cup asparagus spears

- 1 small sweet potato, baked

- 1 tbsp olive oil

- 1 tsp lemon juice

- 1 tsp dried dill

Bake salmon at 400°F for 12-15 minutes. Steam asparagus. Serve with baked sweet potato, drizzle with olive oil and lemon juice, sprinkle with dill.

Macronutrients: 420 calories, 30g carbs, 20g fat, 35g protein

Day 12

Breakfast: Oatmeal with Almonds and Dried Cranberries

Recipe:

- 1/2 cup rolled oats

- 1 cup unsweetened almond milk

- 2 tbsp sliced almonds

- 2 tbsp dried cranberries

- 1 tsp honey

Cook oats with almond milk, top with almonds and cranberries, drizzle with honey.

Macronutrients: 340 calories, 50g carbs, 12g fat, 10g protein

Lunch: Mediterranean Chickpea Salad

Recipe:

- 1/2 cup chickpeas

- 1 cup mixed salad greens

- 1/4 cup cucumber, diced

- 1/4 cup cherry tomatoes, halved

- 1 oz feta cheese

- 1 tbsp olive oil

- 1 tsp lemon juice

Mix all ingredients, dress with olive oil and lemon juice.

Macronutrients: 320 calories, 30g carbs, 18g fat, 15g protein

Dinner: Turkey Meatballs with Zucchini Noodles

Recipe:

- 4 oz ground turkey

- 1 cup zucchini noodles

- 1/4 cup tomato sauce

- 1 tbsp grated Parmesan cheese

- 1 tsp olive oil

- 1 tsp dried basil

Form turkey into meatballs, bake at 375°F for 20 minutes. Sauté zucchini noodles in olive oil, top with tomato sauce and meatballs. Sprinkle with Parmesan and basil.

Macronutrients: 350 calories, 15g carbs, 18g fat, 35g protein

Day 13

Breakfast: Spinach and Mushroom Frittata

Recipe:

- 2 eggs

- 1/4 cup spinach, chopped

- 1/4 cup mushrooms, sliced

- 1 oz goat cheese

- 1 tsp olive oil

Sauté mushrooms, add spinach. Beat eggs, pour over vegetables, add goat cheese, and bake at 350°F for 15 minutes.

Macronutrients: 250 calories, 5g carbs, 18g fat, 20g protein

Lunch: Lentil and Vegetable Soup

Recipe:

- 1/2 cup cooked lentils

- 1 cup mixed vegetables (carrots, celery, onions)

- 2 cups low-sodium vegetable broth

- 1 tsp olive oil

- 1 clove garlic, minced

- 1 tsp dried thyme

Sauté vegetables in olive oil, add garlic and thyme. Add lentils and broth, simmer until vegetables are tender.

Macronutrients: 250 calories, 40g carbs, 5g fat, 15g protein

Dinner: Grilled Cod with Quinoa and Roasted Brussels Sprouts

Recipe:

- 4 oz cod fillet

- 1/2 cup cooked quinoa

- 1 cup Brussels sprouts, halved

- 1 tbsp olive oil

- 1 tsp lemon juice

- 1 tsp dried dill

Grill cod, roast Brussels sprouts with olive oil at 400°F for 20 minutes. Serve with quinoa, drizzle with lemon juice and sprinkle with dill.

Macronutrients: 380 calories, 35g carbs, 12g fat, 35g protein

Day 14

Breakfast: Whole Grain Toast with Almond Butter and Banana

Recipe:

- 2 slices whole grain bread

- 2 tbsp almond butter

- 1 small banana, sliced

- 1 tsp chia seeds

Toast bread, spread almond butter, top with banana slices and chia seeds.

Macronutrients: 420 calories, 55g carbs, 20g fat, 15g protein

Lunch: Greek Salad with Grilled Chicken

Recipe:

- 4 oz grilled chicken breast

- 2 cups mixed salad greens

- 1/4 cup cucumber, diced

- 1/4 cup cherry tomatoes, halved

- 2 tbsp olives, sliced

- 1 oz feta cheese

- 1 tbsp olive oil

- 1 tsp red wine vinegar

Grill chicken, mix all ingredients, dress with olive oil and red wine vinegar.

Macronutrients: 380 calories, 10g carbs, 20g fat, 40g protein

Dinner: Vegetarian Stuffed Bell Peppers

Recipe:

- 1 large bell pepper

- 1/4 cup cooked quinoa

- 1/4 cup black beans

- 1/4 cup corn

- 1/4 cup diced tomatoes

- 1 oz shredded cheddar cheese

- 1 tsp olive oil

- 1 tsp cumin

Mix quinoa, beans, corn, and tomatoes. Stuff into bell pepper, top with cheese. Bake at 375°F for 25 minutes.

Macronutrients: 350 calories, 45g carbs, 12g fat, 20g protein

Day 15

Breakfast: Smoked Salmon and Avocado Toast

Recipe:

- 1 slice whole grain bread

- 1/4 avocado, mashed

- 2 oz smoked salmon

- 1 tsp capers

- 1 tsp lemon juice

Toast bread, spread with mashed avocado. Top with smoked salmon, capers, and a squeeze of lemon juice.

Macronutrients: 280 calories, 20g carbs, 15g fat, 20g protein

Lunch: Quinoa and Roasted Vegetable Bowl

Recipe:

- 1/2 cup cooked quinoa

- 1 cup mixed roasted vegetables (broccoli, cauliflower, carrots)

- 1/4 cup chickpeas

- 1 tbsp tahini

- 1 tsp olive oil

- 1 tsp lemon juice

Roast vegetables with olive oil. Serve over quinoa with chickpeas, drizzle with tahini and lemon juice.

Macronutrients: 350 calories, 50g carbs, 15g fat, 12g protein

Dinner: Herb-Baked Chicken with Sweet Potato and Green Beans

Recipe:

- 4 oz chicken breast

- 1 small sweet potato, cubed

- 1 cup green beans

- 1 tbsp olive oil

- 1 tsp dried rosemary

- 1 tsp dried thyme

Rub chicken with herbs, bake at 375°F for 25 minutes. Roast sweet potato and green beans with olive oil.

Macronutrients: 380 calories, 30g carbs, 12g fat, 35g protein

Day 16

Breakfast: Greek Yogurt Parfait with Berries and Nuts

Recipe:

- 1 cup Greek yogurt

- 1/4 cup mixed berries

- 2 tbsp chopped walnuts

- 1 tsp honey

Layer yogurt with berries and walnuts, drizzle with honey.

Macronutrients: 320 calories, 25g carbs, 18g fat, 25g protein

Lunch: Tuna and White Bean Salad

Recipe:

- 3 oz canned tuna in water, drained

- 1/4 cup white beans

- 1 cup mixed salad greens

- 1/4 cup cherry tomatoes, halved

- 1 tbsp olive oil

- 1 tsp lemon juice

Mix all ingredients, dress with olive oil and lemon juice.

Macronutrients: 320 calories, 20g carbs, 15g fat, 35g protein

Dinner: Grilled Tofu Stir-Fry with Brown Rice

Recipe:

- 4 oz firm tofu, cubed

- 1 cup mixed vegetables (bell peppers, broccoli, carrots)

- 1/2 cup cooked brown rice

- 1 tbsp low-sodium soy sauce

- 1 tsp sesame oil

- 1 clove garlic, minced

Grill tofu, stir-fry vegetables with garlic. Serve over brown rice, drizzle with soy sauce and sesame oil.

Macronutrients: 380 calories, 45g carbs, 15g fat, 20g protein

Day 17

Breakfast: Spinach and Mushroom Omelet

Recipe:

- 2 eggs

- 1/4 cup spinach, chopped

- 1/4 cup mushrooms, sliced

- 1 oz feta cheese

- 1 tsp olive oil

Sauté mushrooms, add spinach. Beat eggs, pour over vegetables, add feta, and fold.

Macronutrients: 250 calories, 5g carbs, 18g fat, 20g protein

Lunch: Lentil and Kale Soup

Recipe:

- 1/2 cup cooked lentils

- 1 cup kale, chopped

- 1/4 cup diced carrots

- 1/4 cup diced onions

- 2 cups low-sodium vegetable broth

- 1 tsp olive oil

- 1 clove garlic, minced

Sauté vegetables in olive oil, add lentils, broth, and garlic. Simmer, add kale before serving.

Macronutrients: 280 calories, 45g carbs, 6g fat, 18g protein

Dinner: Baked Salmon with Quinoa and Asparagus

Recipe:

- 4 oz salmon fillet

- 1/2 cup cooked quinoa

- 1 cup asparagus spears

- 1 tbsp olive oil

- 1 tsp lemon juice

- 1 tsp dried dill

Bake salmon at 400°F for 12-15 minutes. Steam asparagus. Serve with quinoa, drizzle with olive oil and lemon juice, sprinkle with dill.

Macronutrients: 420 calories, 30g carbs, 20g fat, 35g protein

Day 18

Breakfast: Whole Grain Pancakes with Blueberries

Recipe:

- 1/2 cup whole grain pancake mix

- 1/4 cup blueberries

- 1 egg

- 1/4 cup almond milk

- 1 tsp coconut oil

Mix pancake batter, fold in blueberries. Cook in coconut oil.

Macronutrients: 350 calories, 45g carbs, 15g fat, 12g protein

Lunch: Mediterranean Chickpea Salad

Recipe:

- 1/2 cup chickpeas

- 1 cup mixed salad greens

- 1/4 cup cucumber, diced

- 1/4 cup cherry tomatoes, halved

- 1 oz feta cheese

- 1 tbsp olive oil

- 1 tsp lemon juice

Mix all ingredients, dress with olive oil and lemon juice.

Macronutrients: 320 calories, 30g carbs, 18g fat, 15g protein

Dinner: Turkey Meatballs with Zucchini Noodles

Recipe:

- 4 oz ground turkey

- 1 cup zucchini noodles

- 1/4 cup tomato sauce

- 1 tbsp grated Parmesan cheese

- 1 tsp olive oil

- 1 tsp dried basil

Form turkey into meatballs, bake at 375°F for 20 minutes. Sauté zucchini noodles in olive oil, top with tomato sauce and meatballs. Sprinkle with Parmesan and basil.

Macronutrients: 350 calories, 15g carbs, 18g fat, 35g protein

Day 19

Breakfast: Avocado Toast with Poached Egg

Recipe:

- 1 slice whole grain bread

- 1/4 avocado, mashed

- 1 poached egg

- 1 tsp olive oil

- Pinch of red pepper flakes

Toast bread, spread with mashed avocado. Top with poached egg, drizzle with olive oil and sprinkle with red pepper flakes.

Macronutrients: 280 calories, 20g carbs, 18g fat, 12g protein

Lunch: Grilled Chicken and Quinoa Bowl

Recipe:

- 4 oz grilled chicken breast

- 1/2 cup cooked quinoa

- 1/2 cup roasted vegetables (zucchini, eggplant)

- 1 tbsp hummus

- 1 tsp olive oil

Grill chicken, serve over quinoa with roasted vegetables. Top with hummus and drizzle with olive oil.

Macronutrients: 400 calories, 30g carbs, 15g fat, 40g protein

Dinner: Baked Cod with Sweet Potato and Brussels Sprouts

Recipe:

- 4 oz cod fillet

- 1 small sweet potato, cubed

- 1 cup Brussels sprouts, halved

- 1 tbsp olive oil

- 1 tsp lemon juice

- 1 tsp dried dill

Bake cod at 400°F for 12-15 minutes. Roast sweet potato and Brussels sprouts with olive oil. Drizzle with lemon juice and sprinkle with dill.

Macronutrients: 380 calories, 35g carbs, 12g fat, 35g protein

Day 20

Breakfast: Overnight Oats with Chia Seeds and Berries

Recipe:

- 1/2 cup rolled oats

- 1 cup unsweetened almond milk

- 1 tbsp chia seeds

- 1/4 cup mixed berries

- 1 tsp honey

Mix oats, almond milk, and chia seeds. Refrigerate overnight. Top with berries and honey before serving.

Macronutrients: 320 calories, 50g carbs, 10g fat, 10g protein

Lunch: Spinach and Feta Stuffed Chicken Breast

Recipe:

- 4 oz chicken breast

- 1/4 cup spinach, chopped

- 1 oz feta cheese

- 1 cup mixed salad greens

- 1 tbsp olive oil

- 1 tsp balsamic vinegar

Stuff chicken with spinach and feta, bake at 375°F for 25 minutes. Serve with salad dressed with olive oil and balsamic vinegar.

Macronutrients: 350 calories, 5g carbs, 20g fat, 40g protein

Dinner: Vegetarian Chili with Brown Rice

Recipe:

- 1/2 cup mixed beans (kidney, black beans)

- 1/4 cup diced tomatoes

- 1/4 cup diced bell peppers

- 1/4 cup diced onions

- 1/2 cup cooked brown rice

- 1 tsp olive oil

- 1 tsp chili powder

Sauté vegetables in olive oil, add beans, tomatoes, and chili powder. Simmer for 20 minutes. Serve over brown rice.

Macronutrients: 380 calories, 70g carbs, 6g fat, 18g protein

Day 21

Breakfast: Greek Yogurt with Walnuts and Honey

Recipe:

- 1 cup Greek yogurt

- 2 tbsp chopped walnuts

- 1 tsp honey

- 1/4 cup sliced strawberries

Mix yogurt with walnuts and honey, top with strawberries.

Macronutrients: 300 calories, 20g carbs, 15g fat, 25g protein

Lunch: Tuna and Avocado Wrap

Recipe:

- 1 whole wheat tortilla

- 3 oz canned tuna in water, drained

- 1/4 avocado, mashed

- 1 cup mixed salad greens

- 1 tbsp Greek yogurt

- 1 tsp lemon juice

Mix tuna with Greek yogurt and lemon juice. Spread avocado on tortilla, add tuna mixture and greens, roll up.

Macronutrients: 350 calories, 30g carbs, 15g fat, 30g protein

Dinner: Grilled Tofu with Stir-Fried Vegetables and Brown Rice

Recipe:

- 4 oz firm tofu

- 1 cup mixed vegetables (broccoli, carrots, snap peas)

- 1/2 cup cooked brown rice

- 1 tbsp low-sodium soy sauce

- 1 tsp sesame oil

- 1 clove garlic, minced

Grill tofu, stir-fry vegetables with garlic. Serve over brown rice, drizzle with soy sauce and sesame oil.

Macronutrients: 380 calories, 45g carbs, 15g fat, 20g protein

Day 22

Breakfast: Salmon and Spinach Frittata

Recipe:

- 2 eggs

- 2 oz smoked salmon, chopped

- 1/4 cup spinach, chopped

- 1 oz goat cheese

- 1 tsp olive oil

Sauté spinach in olive oil, add beaten eggs and salmon. Top with goat cheese and bake at 350°F for 15 minutes.

Macronutrients: 320 calories, 5g carbs, 22g fat, 30g protein

Lunch: Lentil and Vegetable Soup

Recipe:

- 1/2 cup cooked lentils

- 1 cup mixed vegetables (carrots, celery, onions)

- 2 cups low-sodium vegetable broth

- 1 tsp olive oil

- 1 clove garlic, minced

- 1 tsp dried thyme

Sauté vegetables in olive oil, add garlic and thyme. Add lentils and broth, simmer until vegetables are tender.

Macronutrients: 250 calories, 40g carbs, 5g fat, 15g protein

Dinner: Grilled Chicken with Quinoa and Roasted Brussels Sprouts

Recipe:

- 4 oz chicken breast

- 1/2 cup cooked quinoa

- 1 cup Brussels sprouts, halved

- 1 tbsp olive oil

- 1 tsp balsamic vinegar

- 1 tsp dried rosemary

Grill chicken. Roast Brussels sprouts with olive oil at 400°F for 20 minutes. Serve with quinoa, drizzle with balsamic vinegar and sprinkle with rosemary.

Macronutrients: 400 calories, 35g carbs, 15g fat, 40g protein

Day 23

Breakfast: Blueberry Almond Smoothie Bowl

Recipe:

- 1 cup unsweetened almond milk

- 1/2 cup frozen blueberries

- 1/2 banana

- 1 tbsp almond butter

- 1 tbsp chia seeds

Blend all ingredients except chia seeds. Pour into bowl and top with chia seeds.

Macronutrients: 300 calories, 40g carbs, 15g fat, 8g protein

Lunch: Greek Salad with Grilled Tofu

Recipe:

- 4 oz grilled tofu, cubed

- 2 cups mixed salad greens

- 1/4 cup cucumber, diced

- 1/4 cup cherry tomatoes, halved

- 2 tbsp olives, sliced

- 1 oz feta cheese

- 1 tbsp olive oil

- 1 tsp red wine vinegar

Grill tofu, mix all ingredients, dress with olive oil and red wine vinegar.

Macronutrients: 350 calories, 15g carbs, 25g fat, 25g protein

Dinner: Baked Cod with Sweet Potato Mash and Asparagus

Recipe:

- 4 oz cod fillet

- 1 small sweet potato, mashed

- 1 cup asparagus spears

- 1 tbsp olive oil

- 1 tsp lemon juice

- 1 tsp dried dill

Bake cod at 400°F for 12-15 minutes. Steam asparagus. Serve with mashed sweet potato, drizzle with olive oil and lemon juice, sprinkle with dill.

Macronutrients: 380 calories, 35g carbs, 12g fat, 35g protein

Day 24

Breakfast: Whole Grain Toast with Avocado and Poached Egg

Recipe:

- 1 slice whole grain bread

- 1/4 avocado, mashed

- 1 poached egg

- 1 tsp olive oil

- Pinch of red pepper flakes

Toast bread, spread with mashed avocado. Top with poached egg, drizzle with olive oil and sprinkle with red pepper flakes.

Macronutrients: 280 calories, 20g carbs, 18g fat, 12g protein

Lunch: Chickpea and Vegetable Curry

Recipe:

- 1/2 cup chickpeas

- 1 cup mixed vegetables (cauliflower, peas, carrots)

- 1/4 cup coconut milk

- 1/2 cup cooked brown rice

- 1 tsp curry powder

- 1 tsp olive oil

Sauté vegetables in olive oil, add chickpeas, coconut milk, and curry powder. Simmer and serve over brown rice.

Macronutrients: 400 calories, 60g carbs, 15g fat, 15g protein

Dinner: Grilled Salmon with Quinoa and Roasted Broccoli

Recipe:

- 4 oz salmon fillet

- 1/2 cup cooked quinoa

- 1 cup broccoli florets

- 1 tbsp olive oil

- 1 tsp lemon juice

- 1 tsp dried oregano

Grill salmon, roast broccoli with olive oil at 400°F for 20 minutes. Serve with quinoa, drizzle with lemon juice and sprinkle with oregano.

Macronutrients: 420 calories, 30g carbs, 20g fat, 35g protein

Day 25

Breakfast: Oatmeal with Walnuts and Cinnamon

Recipe:

- 1/2 cup rolled oats

- 1 cup unsweetened almond milk

- 2 tbsp chopped walnuts

- 1 tsp honey

- 1/4 tsp cinnamon

Cook oats with almond milk, top with walnuts, honey, and cinnamon.

Macronutrients: 320 calories, 40g carbs, 15g fat, 10g protein

Lunch: Turkey and Avocado Wrap

Recipe:

- 1 whole wheat tortilla

- 3 oz sliced turkey breast

- 1/4 avocado, sliced

- 1 cup mixed salad greens

- 1 tbsp hummus

Spread hummus on tortilla, add turkey, avocado, and greens. Roll and slice.

Macronutrients: 350 calories, 30g carbs, 15g fat, 25g protein

Dinner: Baked Trout with Roasted Vegetables

Recipe:

- 4 oz trout fillet

- 1 cup mixed vegetables (zucchini, bell peppers, onions)

- 1/2 cup cooked quinoa

- 1 tbsp olive oil

- 1 tsp lemon juice

- 1 tsp dried thyme

Bake trout at 400°F for 12-15 minutes. Roast vegetables with olive oil. Serve with quinoa, drizzle with lemon juice and sprinkle with thyme.

Macronutrients: 400 calories, 30g carbs, 18g fat, 35g protein

Day 26

Breakfast: Greek Yogurt Parfait

Recipe:

- 1 cup Greek yogurt

- 1/4 cup granola

- 1/2 cup mixed berries

- 1 tbsp chia seeds

Layer yogurt, granola, berries, and chia seeds in a glass.

Macronutrients: 340 calories, 35g carbs, 12g fat, 25g protein

Lunch: Lentil and Spinach Salad

Recipe:

- 1/2 cup cooked lentils

- 2 cups spinach

- 1/4 cup cherry tomatoes, halved

- 1 oz feta cheese

- 1 tbsp olive oil

- 1 tsp balsamic vinegar

Mix all ingredients, dress with olive oil and balsamic vinegar.

Macronutrients: 300 calories, 30g carbs, 15g fat, 18g protein

Dinner: Grilled Tofu Steak with Sweet Potato and Green Beans

Recipe:

- 4 oz firm tofu, sliced

- 1 small sweet potato, cubed

- 1 cup green beans

- 1 tbsp olive oil

- 1 tsp soy sauce

- 1 tsp sesame seeds

Grill tofu, roast sweet potato and green beans with olive oil. Drizzle with soy sauce and sprinkle with sesame seeds.

Macronutrients: 380 calories, 45g carbs, 18g fat, 20g protein

Day 27

Breakfast: Spinach and Mushroom Omelet

Recipe:

- 2 eggs

- 1/4 cup spinach, chopped

- 1/4 cup mushrooms, sliced

- 1 oz goat cheese

- 1 tsp olive oil

Sauté mushrooms, add spinach. Beat eggs, pour over vegetables, add goat cheese, and fold.

Macronutrients: 250 calories, 5g carbs, 18g fat, 20g protein

Lunch: Quinoa and Chickpea Bowl

Recipe:

- 1/2 cup cooked quinoa

- 1/4 cup chickpeas

- 1 cup mixed roasted vegetables (broccoli, carrots, onions)

- 1 tbsp tahini

- 1 tsp lemon juice

Mix all ingredients, dress with tahini and lemon juice.

Macronutrients: 350 calories, 50g carbs, 12g fat, 15g protein

Dinner: Baked Chicken with Asparagus and Brown Rice

Recipe:

- 4 oz chicken breast

- 1 cup asparagus spears

- 1/2 cup cooked brown rice

- 1 tbsp olive oil

- 1 tsp dried rosemary

- 1 tsp lemon zest

Bake chicken at 375°F for 25 minutes. Roast asparagus with olive oil. Serve with brown rice, sprinkle with rosemary and lemon zest.

Macronutrients: 400 calories, 35g carbs, 12g fat, 40g protein

Day 28

Breakfast: Avocado Toast with Smoked Salmon

Recipe:

- 1 slice whole grain bread

- 1/4 avocado, mashed

- 2 oz smoked salmon

- 1 tsp capers

- 1 tsp lemon juice

Toast bread, spread with mashed avocado. Top with smoked salmon, capers, and a squeeze of lemon juice.

Macronutrients: 280 calories, 20g carbs, 15g fat, 20g protein

Lunch: Mediterranean Vegetable Soup

Recipe:

- 1 cup mixed vegetables (zucchini, tomatoes, bell peppers)

- 1/4 cup white beans

- 2 cups low-sodium vegetable broth

- 1 tsp olive oil

- 1 clove garlic, minced

- 1 tsp dried oregano

Sauté vegetables and garlic in olive oil, add beans, broth, and oregano. Simmer until vegetables are tender.

Macronutrients: 200 calories, 30g carbs, 5g fat, 10g protein

Dinner: Grilled Salmon with Quinoa and Roasted Brussels Sprouts

Recipe:

- 4 oz salmon fillet

- 1/2 cup cooked quinoa

- 1 cup Brussels sprouts, halved

- 1 tbsp olive oil

- 1 tsp lemon juice

- 1 tsp dried dill

Grill salmon, roast Brussels sprouts with olive oil at 400°F for 20 minutes. Serve with quinoa, drizzle with lemon juice and sprinkle with dill.

Macronutrients: 420 calories, 30g carbs, 20g fat, 35g protein

I apologize for the oversight. You're absolutely right, and I thank you for bringing this to my attention. Let me provide you with the meal plans for days 29 and 30 to complete the 30-day plan.

Day 29

Breakfast: Blueberry Almond Smoothie

Recipe:

- 1 cup unsweetened almond milk

- 1/2 cup frozen blueberries

- 1 tbsp almond butter

- 1 tbsp chia seeds

- 1/2 scoop vanilla protein powder (optional)

Blend all ingredients until smooth.

Macronutrients: 280 calories, 25g carbs, 16g fat, 15g protein

Lunch: Tuna and White Bean Salad

Recipe:

- 3 oz canned tuna in water, drained

- 1/4 cup white beans

- 1 cup mixed salad greens

- 1/4 cup cherry tomatoes, halved

- 1 tbsp olive oil

- 1 tsp lemon juice

Mix all ingredients, dress with olive oil and lemon juice.

Macronutrients: 320 calories, 20g carbs, 15g fat, 35g protein

Dinner: Herb-Roasted Chicken with Quinoa and Roasted Vegetables

Recipe:

- 4 oz chicken breast

- 1/2 cup cooked quinoa

- 1 cup mixed roasted vegetables (broccoli, carrots, red onion)

- 1 tbsp olive oil

- 1 tsp dried herbs (rosemary, thyme, oregano)

Roast chicken and vegetables with herbs and olive oil. Serve with quinoa.

Macronutrients: 400 calories, 30g carbs, 15g fat, 40g protein

Day 30

Breakfast: Spinach and Feta Omelet

Recipe:

- 2 eggs

- 1/4 cup spinach, chopped

- 1 oz feta cheese

- 1 tsp olive oil

Cook omelet with spinach and feta in olive oil.

Macronutrients: 250 calories, 5g carbs, 18g fat, 20g protein

Lunch: Mediterranean Chickpea Salad

Recipe:

- 1/2 cup chickpeas

- 1 cup mixed salad greens

- 1/4 cup cucumber, diced

- 1/4 cup cherry tomatoes, halved

- 1 oz feta cheese

- 1 tbsp olive oil

- 1 tsp lemon juice

Mix all ingredients, dress with olive oil and lemon juice.

Macronutrients: 320 calories, 30g carbs, 18g fat, 15g protein

Dinner: Grilled Salmon with Sweet Potato and Asparagus

Recipe:

- 4 oz salmon fillet

- 1 small sweet potato, baked

- 1 cup asparagus spears

- 1 tbsp olive oil

- 1 tsp lemon juice

- 1 tsp dried dill

Grill salmon, roast asparagus. Serve with baked sweet potato, drizzle with olive oil and lemon juice, sprinkle with dill.

Macronutrients: 420 calories, 30g carbs, 20g fat, 35g protein

Summary of the Key Nutritional Aspects Of This 30-Day Meal Plan Designed For Brain Health in Individuals Over 60

1. Omega-3 Fatty Acids: The plan includes frequent servings of fatty fish like salmon, trout, and cod, which are rich in omega-3 fatty acids, particularly DHA, essential for brain health.

2. Antioxidants: Abundant colorful fruits and vegetables (berries, leafy greens, bell peppers) provide antioxidants that combat oxidative stress and inflammation in the brain.

3. Whole Grains: The plan incorporates whole grains like quinoa, brown rice, and whole grain bread, providing steady energy and B vitamins for cognitive function.

4. Lean Proteins: A variety of lean protein sources (fish, poultry, legumes, tofu) support neurotransmitter production and overall brain health.

5. Healthy Fats: Includes sources of monounsaturated and polyunsaturated fats from avocados, nuts, seeds, and olive oil, which support brain cell structure and function.

6. Low in Added Sugars: The meals are naturally sweetened with fruits, limiting added sugars that can contribute to cognitive decline.

7. Hydration: While not explicitly stated in each meal, adequate hydration is assumed and crucial for cognitive function.

8. Variety: The plan offers a diverse range of foods to ensure a wide spectrum of nutrients and to prevent dietary boredom.

9. Portion Control: Meals are balanced and portioned to support a healthy weight, which is important for brain health.

10. Brain-Boosting Herbs and Spices: Incorporates herbs and spices like turmeric, rosemary, and thyme, known for their cognitive benefits.

11. Limited Processed Foods: The focus is on whole, minimally processed foods to reduce intake of unhealthy fats and additives.

12. Balanced Macronutrients: Each meal provides a balance of carbohydrates, proteins, and fats to support overall health and stable blood sugar levels.

This meal plan aims to provide a nutrient-dense, brain-healthy diet that also supports overall health in older adults. It's important to note that individual nutritional needs may vary, and consultation with a healthcare provider or registered dietitian is recommended for personalized advice.

Weekly grocery shopping list for the 30-day HEALTHY Meal Plan

Keep in mind that some items may overlap between weeks, and you may need to adjust quantities based on personal preferences and portion sizes.

Week 1

Produce:

- Blueberries

- Mixed berries

- Bananas

- Lemons

- Avocados

- Cherry tomatoes

- Mixed salad greens

- Spinach

- Kale

- Carrots

- Celery

- Onions

- Garlic

- Broccoli

- Cauliflower

- Bell peppers

- Zucchini

- Asparagus

- Brussels sprouts

- Sweet potatoes

Proteins:

- Salmon

- Chicken breast

- Turkey breast

- Tofu

- Eggs

- Canned tuna (in water)

Dairy and Alternatives:

- Greek yogurt

- Feta cheese

- Unsweetened almond milk

Grains and Legumes:

- Rolled oats

- Quinoa

- Brown rice

- Whole grain bread

- Lentils

- Chickpeas

Nuts and Seeds:

- Walnuts

- Chia seeds

- Almonds

Pantry Items:

- Olive oil

- Balsamic vinegar

- Low-sodium vegetable broth

- Low-sodium soy sauce

- Honey

- Dried herbs (thyme, rosemary, dill, basil)

Week 2

Produce:

- Strawberries

- Mixed berries

- Bananas

- Lemons

- Avocados

- Cherry tomatoes

- Cucumbers

- Mixed salad greens

- Spinach

- Kale

- Carrots

- Onions

- Garlic

- Broccoli

- Bell peppers

- Zucchini

- Eggplant

- Asparagus

- Brussels sprouts

- Sweet potatoes

- Green beans

Proteins:

- Salmon

- Chicken breast

- Ground turkey

- Tofu

- Eggs

- Canned tuna (in water)

Dairy and Alternatives:

- Greek yogurt

- Feta cheese

- Goat cheese

- Unsweetened almond milk

Grains and Legumes:

- Rolled oats

- Quinoa

- Brown rice

- Whole grain bread

- Whole wheat tortillas

- Lentils

- Chickpeas

- Mixed beans (kidney, black beans)

Nuts and Seeds:

- Walnuts

- Chia seeds

Pantry Items:

- Olive oil

- Balsamic vinegar

- Red wine vinegar

- Low-sodium vegetable broth

- Low-sodium soy sauce

- Tomato sauce

- Dried herbs (thyme, rosemary, dill, basil, oregano)

- Chili powder

- Hummus

Week 3

Produce:

- Blueberries

- Strawberries

- Bananas

- Lemons

- Avocados

- Cherry tomatoes

- Cucumbers

- Mixed salad greens

- Spinach

- Kale

- Carrots

- Celery

- Onions

- Garlic

- Broccoli

- Brussels sprouts

- Bell peppers

- Zucchini

- Asparagus

- Sweet potatoes

- Green beans

- Mushrooms

Proteins:

- Salmon

- Chicken breast

- Tofu

- Eggs

- Canned tuna (in water)

- Smoked salmon

Dairy and Alternatives:

- Greek yogurt

- Feta cheese

- Goat cheese

- Unsweetened almond milk

Grains and Legumes:

- Rolled oats

- Quinoa

- Brown rice

- Whole grain bread

- Whole wheat tortillas

- Lentils

- Chickpeas

Nuts and Seeds:

- Walnuts

- Chia seeds

- Almond butter

Pantry Items:

- Olive oil

- Balsamic vinegar

- Red wine vinegar

- Low-sodium vegetable broth

- Low-sodium soy sauce

- Dried herbs (thyme, rosemary, dill, basil, oregano)

- Coconut milk

- Curry powder

- Honey

Week 4

Produce:

- Mixed berries

- Lemons

- Avocados

- Cherry tomatoes

- Cucumbers

- Mixed salad greens

- Spinach

- Carrots

- Onions

- Garlic

- Broccoli

- Bell peppers

- Zucchini

- Asparagus

- Sweet potatoes

- Green beans

- Mushrooms

- Brussels sprouts

Proteins:

- Salmon

- Chicken breast

- Turkey breast

- Tofu

- Eggs

- Smoked salmon

- Trout

Dairy and Alternatives:

- Greek yogurt

- Feta cheese

- Goat cheese

- Unsweetened almond milk

Grains and Legumes:

- Rolled oats

- Quinoa

- Brown rice

- Whole grain bread

- Whole wheat tortillas

- Lentils

- Chickpeas

- White beans

Nuts and Seeds:

- Walnuts

- Chia seeds

- Sesame seeds

Pantry Items:

- Olive oil

- Balsamic vinegar

- Low-sodium vegetable broth

- Low-sodium soy sauce

- Dried herbs (thyme, rosemary, dill, oregano)

- Granola

- Capers

- Tahini

- Honey

- Cinnamon

Remember to adjust quantities based on your specific needs and any leftover ingredients from previous weeks. Also, check your pantry before shopping to avoid buying duplicates of items you may already have. Lastly, feel free to make substitutions based on personal preferences or seasonal availability of produce.

For Information and Health Tips, Please follow on Instagram: @PlatinumFitAP

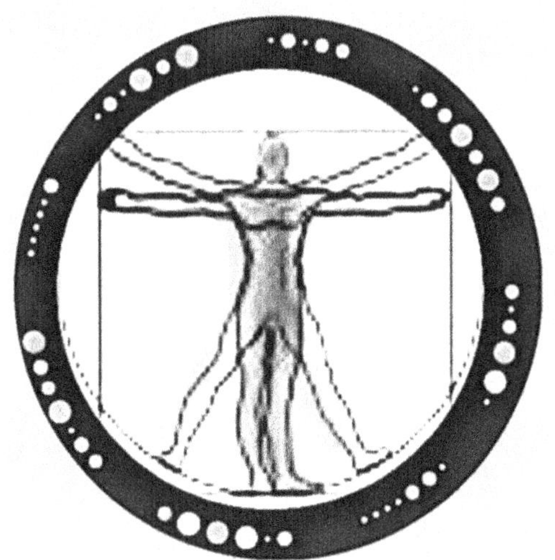